BILLY BARNETT

HEALTHY ADULT

The Essential Guide Towards a Healthier and Fitter You, Discover the Step-by-Step Approach On How You Can Achieve A Healthier Body and Mind You Can Be Proud Of!

Descrierea CIP a Bibliotecii Naţionale a României
BILLY BARNETT
   HEALTHY ADULT. The Essential Guide Towards a
Healthier and Fitter You, Discover the Step-by-Step Approach On
How You Can Achieve A Healthier Body and Mind You Can Be
Proud Of! / Billy Barnett. – Bucharest: Editura My Ebook, 2020
   ISBN

BILLY BARNETT

HEALTHY ADULT

The Essential Guide Towards a Healthier and Fitter You, Discover the Step-by-Step Approach On How You Can Achieve A Healthier Body and Mind You Can Be Proud Of!

My Ebook Publishing House
Bucharest, 2020

TABLE OF CONTENTS

WHY HEALTH MATTERS

It's no secret that a healthy lifestyle is beneficial for everyone. Creating a positive mental state, making healthy food choices, and partaking in regular physical activity are all major factors to your overall well-being. When you can maintain a balanced life that includes a healthy mind, body and soul, you'll find that the external events of your life – all that stuff you can't control – have much less effect on your happiness and success in life.

Your health does not just make your body look better and help to ward off disease and disorders, it provides a solid foundation to the reality that you can create a better life and it doesn't have anything to do with what is happening outside of you.

Taking control of your health is most effective when you take a look at yourself with a holistic perspective. The holistic approach to health takes into account the complete person; their physical, psychological and social needs which directly relate to their spiritual selves. Basically, you would improve your overall well-being by integrating aspects of every part of yourself and by not just eating right and getting exercise. Your mind needs stimulation, you need social interaction and solid relationships, and you need to nurture your spiritual side along with honoring the operation of your body's physical aspects.

When someone desires to improve their health there is always a much more long-term commitment when they have made a whole lifestyle change rather than just deciding to try a new diet for 2 weeks. You really shouldn't restrict foods or participate in a rigorous exercise regime for short periods of time. Although it seems to be a popular trend to try out the next new diet or be part of the next 'exercise craze', it isn't these short bursts of diet and exercise changes that provide lasting health benefits. You will be much better served by taking the time and effort to truly look at your whole self; preparing yourself mentally, gaining lots of knowledge about healthy living, gradually adding positive habits and slowly eliminating harmful habits, and discovering ways to nurture your inner self as well.

As you're looking at the areas of your life involving food and exercise,don't leave out a vital component of a complete life – your spiritual health.

Nurturing your mind, body and spirit is a package deal. You can't connect with your true self and commit to a renewed life of health without nourishing your spiritual side.

5 TIPS TO A HEALTHY SPIRITUAL LIFE

We are all on a journey in this life to do great things. These great things are big and small and can have an effect on millions of people or just one person. It is a lifelong quest to figure out what your life purpose is.

Discovering what really motivates you and gives you the energy to be always growing is part of your spiritual path. It doesn't matter what religion you follow or where your beliefs lie, there are certain elements to focus on to find your place and discover what significance your life plays in the world around you.

Your inner growth is the most important growth in your life, not only because it's what forms your perspective (which gives you a positive or negative take on your surroundings), but also because it is how you will discover what you were created for. There's nothing more peaceful than knowing that you're living your life the way you were designed to. The five points below are what you need to focus on to live a life of purpose and meaning:

1. **Have faith in your personal power**. This can be related to one's faith in a specific religion, but faith is not limited to religion. Believe that you have been given special qualities and that there is a universal source that connects one to all. Believe that you are capable of doing great and satisfying things and that you'll get through all those ups and downs in life. The most important things have to be believed to be seen.

2. **Have patience in your wait for the right things at the right time**. Patience is a virtue and not easily come by, which makes for lots of opportunities to grow in this area. We want things right when we think of them. Instant gratification is mainstream in society and it seems that it should be that way in our spiritual life, but unfortunately we're not here to make the rules, we're here to discover 'the good life'

3. **Generate love continuously and about everything**. To love under any circumstances really is the greatest achievement of all and it's really not that hard once you have a few years of practice under your belt. Love does make the world

work right and feeling love in difficult situations will make your inner world a much happier place; love for yourself and others.

4. **Develop a prayer practice**. Don't worry about all those rules out there about how to pray. You just need to have the intention to connect with your creator and be aware of what you're thankful for, what you'd like in your life and what you'd like for others. Say it out loud, think it, or even write it down in your very own prayer journal. Just put it out in the universe and take comfort that you've been heard.

5. **Be aware of creation**. Nature is all around us, providing, nurturing, and sharing. Take time to spend quiet moments in natural surroundings and be aware of how perfectly nature lives. You'll soon strengthen your faith in the gifts and abilities that have been given to you to live a truly blessed life.

Living a happy life has very little to do with what goes on around you and a whole lot to do with how you perceive the world around you. To help your thoughts stay positive grow your faith, patience, love, prayer and belief in a faithful creation. You have been created for great things and it's up to you to act on those qualities you have been blessed with.

With an inquisitive motivation and a genuine believe in the reality of a healthier you, start off your journey to better health with this checklist of a healthy life. There are various benefits to healthy living, some of which you will likely be aware of and some that you will be comforted to know will be a reward of your step in the right direction.

A Healthy Life Checklist:

- ✓ A positive attitude about life and living
- ✓ An open mind to new and nurturing activities
- ✓ Less (or no) negative reactions and more control of emotions
- ✓ General benefits of physical activity such as increased energy, better muscle tone, improved metabolism and greater flexibility
- ✓ More productive and effective in personal and professional activities
- ✓ Additional years of living a better quality of life
- ✓ Reduced risk of chronic illness
- ✓ Aspirations to achieve more in all areas of life
- ✓ Reduced occurrence of bone loss associated with ageing
- ✓ Improved mood and self-esteem

✓ Better functioning of all body systems

With all that is gained from leading a healthy life you can be assured that it is well worth the initial effort of making the gradual shift to better living.

Slowly but surely you can make all the changes necessary in different areas of your life to get the most out each day with a renewed optimism that is sure to infect the people around you. So don't just make the lifestyle change for yourself – do it for your children, your spouse, your parents, siblings, friends and even those casual acquaintances that will be inspired to take a closer look at their way of living when they see how full of life you are when you choose to put health first.

Below are a few inspiring words to encourage you to live a healthier way:

"A vigorous five-mile walk will do more good for an unhappy but otherwise healthy adult than all the medicine and psychology in the world."

Paul Dudley White (1886-1973) American physician and cardiologist.

"Those who do not find time for exercise will have to find time for illness."

Edward Smith-Stanley (1752-1834) English statesman and Prime Minister of the United Kingdom

He who takes medicine and neglects his diet wastes the skill of his doctors.

Chinese Proverb

Just because you're not sick doesn't mean you're healthy.

Good health is not to be taken for granted. Yet, until it's in jeopardy it's not regarded as a top priority. A sluggish body and a few extra pounds isn't a major cause for concern, but it is a sign that improvements could be made. Getting informed by reading this book is an indication that you are aware that health matters and you want to learn about a healthier way to live.

Whether you've already being working at improving in the area of nutrition and exercise or this is your first real introduction to a healthier way of life you'll gain lots of knowledge and practical advice.

DEVELOPING A HEALTHY MINDSET

While you won't find too many people saying that they don't understand why being healthy is better, you will find many people admitting that changing their habits is too hard to do. Unfortunately, you can't avoid the hard part of altering a way of life that consists of well-ingrained habits. You can find comfort in knowing that anything that is truly worth doing is a struggle, and it is that struggle that will make you improve on the inside and out.

Change is constant. Are you going to have control over some of that change?

Determination, self-motivation, and beginning with the end in mind will get you on your way to a healthier life. It really is all in your head – *well…* what internalizes the need for change and the motivation to keep on track is all in your head – in your mind to be exact. The power of your mind can make or break your success in anything you aspire to achieve. Achieving a healthier way of life is no different.

Knowledge is Power

The first and most important step to getting in the right mindset is to arm yourself with knowledge and support. There is a wealth of information available on how and why to lead a healthier life and you need to soak in as much as possible. There are a number of different methods for effective information gathering. Depending on your preferences, you will find some or all of the options helpful on the following list:

Search the internet for any information about: leading a healthier life (search *'healthy living tips' 'making healthy changes')*, understanding the resistance to change (search *'breaking bad habits' 'why it's hard to change'*), and connecting with others that are working towards a healthier lifestyle (search *"health forums", "health boards"*)

Find a couple of books that you can study to be well equipped with facts and tips for a health-focused lifestyle. The best type of book for this method is one that doesn't necessarily need to be read from beginning to end and has tidbits of information as opposed the pages of paragraphs. Highlight sections and bookmark pages that are of special interest to you and really make the book your own by writing in notes about your thoughts and experience with the content of the book. Some examples of appropriate books are:

The 150 Most Effective Ways to Boost Your Energy by Jonny Bowden

500 of the Most Important Health Tips You'll Ever Need by Hazel Courteney

Record your thoughts and motivation to having a healthier life in your personal health journal or in a blog. Posting your healthy living thoughts online provides an added accountability factor and allows the openness to be able to connect with others on the issue, which will provide you with lots of new insight and information about the many facets of a healthful motivation.

Watch documentaries and short videos on health issues. Learning through visual elements provides an opportunity to be effected in a way that allows many people to internalize the facts more effectively. If you've got access to Netflix, they have numerous documentaries on health and you can search online for health documentaries and find various films that way.

Get connected to people that are living in a much healthier way than yourself. You are influenced by the people that surround you, so talking with, and spending time with people that are making healthy choices will naturally rub off on you even if you don't have in depth conversations about healthy living.

Get yourself an accountability partner that you will check in with regularly to let them know about your health-focused journey.

Although this could be someone that is already leading a healthy life as mentioned in the point above, this approach is usually more effective if it's someone that is in the same situation as you and you can be each other's accountability partner. It is so much more motivating to be checking in with someone that is in the same boat and you look to each other for support. This could be a great opportunity to assist someone in your life to go for a healthier lifestyle and be supporting them as much as they will support you.

Develop Your Self-Awareness

Getting your mind in health mode should also involve a self-analysis of your pre-conceived notions about food and your body with the purpose of identifying some of the underlying causes of unhealthy habits and ways to **replace those harmful habits with good habits**. By taking this mental check-in before you really make a lot of changes to your day-to-day activities you can identify potential triggers and problem areas that you will be able to address better when the time comes.

For instance, you may feel that one of your unhealthy food habits is regularly eating at fast food restaurants, which is not the best place to find wholesome food. You identify that it's an easy source of food and since you are not that great in the kitchen, it substitutes for a full meal. To address your well-established habit of fast food eating you can educate yourself on the poor nutritional value and harmful food-like ingredients that are used in fast food and gain some knowledge about the 'slow food' way of eating and how to make some quick meals.

A Closer Look at Leaving Bad Habits Behind

We all look at ourselves time and again and notice the things that we do and say. When we honestly analyze our actions and words we will identify some bad habits that need to go to be able to function at our best. After that first step of noticing what bad habits we'd like to be rid of, we need to take action with our heads held high and our pride in check.

With a bit of persistence and determination you can get rid of those useless and sometimes damaging habits for good. **Be intentional about your actions and be in tune to your desired outcome**...

...a life that you have more control over.

Below are 3 techniques you can use separately or in conjunction with each other to get over your harmful habits that invade every area of your life:

- Replace those bad habits with something that is good. For example, if you find you are talking negative about other people then make a note to yourself that every time you talk bad about someone you have to think of something good about them. Actually write down your intention on paper and either have it posted somewhere you'll see it regularly throughout the day, or carry it around with you in your pocket so you can be reminded of it. There is something good you can say about anyone, even if it's just about their hairstyle or color of their shoes. The point here is to shift your thinking from negative to positive – a much better mindset for everyone!

- Pick one habit that you'd like to be rid of and focus on that one for a week or even a month. Use that power of writing again and write down what you'd like to change, then make small notes *every day* about your progress. You might have days where you're noting that you did the bad habit x number of times that day and you'll have days where you'll realize that you went through the whole day without giving in to the habit at all. The point of this technique is to increase your awareness every day as you're spending a few minutes thinking about how you progressed with 'curbing' this bad habit.

- Enlist your accountability partner. It is quite helpful to know that you are going to have to explain to someone how you're doing with your personal growth. This person that you will be reporting to should not be judging your actions, but merely be a listening ear and a source of encouragement to carry on with your goal. It would be most helpful if you were able to be their source of accountability as well so it evens the level of confidence.

Self-improvement occurs over time and the worst thing you could do is to overwhelm yourself with too much change at once. The most common reason for failure in stopping bad habits is *not* giving it daily attention.

Don't make it lengthy or judgmental, just be aware of what your intentions are and make a casual plan for change. You also need to take action – not just think about change or just write down your ideas for change. We all pick up bad habits here and there and it is a part of life to be aware of what needs to go. Be persistent, be intentional and be positive in the light of a healthier life.

Know Your Stuff Then Strengthen Your Mind

Most people decide they need to make some changes to their life and have lots of ideas about what they want to stop doing and what they want to start doing but don't really prepare themselves for the mental and emotional reaction to this new way of living. Usually they can sustain a week or two of their ideal life, but without the mental preparation they slowly step back into their old routine and before they know it, they've lost all motivation and all progress has been lost.

Has this happened to you?

The trick is to prepare your mind for the inevitable desire to revert back to the old way. Make your new lifestyle aspirations a permanent shift, not just a temporary fad, and spend the time consuming lots of knowledge that encourages healthy changes, connecting with others for support, and determining the areas that you see as potentially difficult in your progress to a better life. Overall, be committed to the eventual outcome of the decision to be healthy; don't take any other outcome than that.

We'll end this chapter with an excerpt from Richard Carlson's book *You Can Feel Good Again*:

"Commitment is a powerful tool for change. It takes pressure off of you by removing the uncertainty that often accompanies a lack of commitment. Marriage, for example, is a commitment. When couples marry, there is a reasonable belief that regardless of what might happen, the commitment will carry the couple through.

Prior to marriage, people often feel insecure about losing their partner, but the commitment relieves their anxiety and gives them the freedom to "let go" of their concerns; it fosters hope.

Without commitment, success in any venture is difficult. Whether you are dieting, studying for an exam, learning to play tennis, starting a project or deciding to be happy, commitment is an important step."

HEALTHIER FUEL: CHANGING YOUR DIET

What you feed your body is the biggest factor in the health of your whole self. Not just your physical self, but also your emotional, social, mental and spiritual self. How the body uses food effects every part of our being so dramatically that if you only take great care in fueling your body with the most appropriate nutrients and avoid all those unnecessary 'filler' foods then you'll achieve an excellent level of health without putting much effort into exercising. That being said, you'll also have a hard time avoiding activity when your body is running on high quality fuel!

You pretty much have to be living under a rock to avoid being regularly bombarded by advertising and association recommendations regarding many foods that are *supposedly* 'healthy' for you. Truth is, the claim of a healthy status shouldn't be taken as a definite benefit to your body. You need to get the facts from unbiased sources to be sure you're getting the most accurate information and advice about what truly is the right combination of nutrients and macronutrients (the protein, fat, and carbohydrates) to supply the optimum performance fuel for your body.

If you're like most people, changing your thinking will be a great benefit to changing your diet and there's only one concept you need to change to ease your way into healthful eating:

Food is not for your emotional pleasure, but a source of fuel to provide your body the needed energy to function properly.

A high-performance car needs high performance fuel that contains only essentials needed for the functioning of the engine. In relation, if your body was to run on high-performance food and not have to process food with little or no nutritional value that merely staves off hunger, then you would discover a whole new body that has every system running so efficiently you would have the overwhelming feeling of being able to achieve anything.

Don't worry though, the novelty of a high-functioning body does wear off and you'll know your limitations within the human body, and you'll do just fine settling for a human body that is at the peak of its ability.

Changing eating habits isn't easy though, so to make changes that stick you'll want to use these tidbits of advice to cement your new way of fueling your body into place.

Keep a record of the food you eat and what you drink for at least a week. This will help you constructively judge your eating habits and identify areas for change, as well as make you accountable for your food choices. Studies have shown this to be one of the vital components to successful diet changes and weight loss.

Eat *s l ow l y* so that you can allow your body the time to signal that you're full and to be much more satisfied by the flavor of the food.

No need to count calories and measure portion sizes. Be more concerned with making food choices that are in their most natural state (vegetable, fruits, grains, pulses, unprocessed meats and much more), and *including a wide range of color and variety.*

It's good to have a long-term plan of how you'd like to be feeding your body, but you'll be most successful if you **make small changes over time**. For example, if you would like to be consuming more vegetables, start by preparing an array of raw vegetables that you have on hand to snack on and make this

28

your main goal for the week. Then the following week, you may want to start creating some dinner recipes that are focused on more healthy ingredients. Little by little you will be building new habits that will stick.

Drink water regularly throughout the day. Not only does water flush toxins and waste products out of the body, it also helps you feel more energetic, gets you thinking more clearly, improves the appearance of your skin and helps you to feel less hungry. *If you're not drinking around 2 litres of water a day, make this one of your first diet changes to implement.*

Moderation is the key to any diet so don't feel like you can never enjoy your favorite sugar-laden treat or enjoy the convenience of fast- food. Just don't make it your regular routine. As well, use the concept of *moderation and balance with portion sizes*. Don't fill your plate with a high-carb portion of pasta and only include a small serving of low-carb vegetables. Although carbohydrates are an important part of a healthy diet, they are often over consumed and not conducive to your body's optimum performance or in managing a healthy weight.

Try not to be eating anything within 4 hours of going to sleep. Studies suggest that this simple dietary change is beneficial for the digestive system and in avoiding the high fat/high calorie snacking that often occurs after the last meal of the day.

Learn to like the good sources of fat. Fat tends to get a bad reputation for being the main instigator of weight gain, but it's really over-consumption (mainly over-consumption of high carbohydrate foods) that cause weight gain and sluggish body processes. *Get well educated on the good sources of fat that are so vital to the nourishment of your body.* Just a couple of excellent options are: nuts & seeds, plant oils, avocados, fish, peanut butter (with just peanuts) and tofu.

Protein is an energy packed element of a balanced diet. It's integral to the building of muscle and gives the body a great energy kick along with other healthful benefits, but there also seems to be a tad too much emphasis on the protein portion of the meal on the average plate, specifically when it comes to meat protein. It's not the protein part of the meat that's the problem though it's what comes along with the protein, which means you should limit red meats and avoid all processed meats. No need to think about taking meat right out of your diet, especially if you enjoy it, but **get familiar with consuming a healthy portion and eating the leanest cuts of unprocessed meat.**

Limit sugar and salt and recognize all the hidden sources of these health threats. Although it can be a given that consuming too much sugar and salt isn't ideal, the biggest hurdle is being informed enough to realize all the places these veiled ingredients are hiding.

For the most part, your food sources are going to start becoming more and more natural but there will still be opportunities for the sugar and salt to sneak their way into your meals without you even realizing it. Keep in mind that salt is commonly used to cure meats and to preserve canned foods and commonly referred to as sodium. The table below reveals some of the alternate terms for sugar:

Sugar Aliases
Dextrose
Fructose
Glucose
Maltose Sucrose
Maltodextrin (dextrin) Brown rice syrup Cane sugar Molasses
Corn sweetener Corn syrup Cane juice
Fruit juice concentrates Barley malt
Caramel

Note: Ingredients that contain any of the above words in them can be considered a sugar product as well.

The Serious Solution to Sinful Snacking

The best way to fuel your body is to be consuming good nutrients throughout the day. With meals generally spaced 4-6 hours apart snacking is a pretty major part of your eating life. Many people, especially adults with busy schedules, will either avoid snacking altogether or snack on the highly-processed, high-sugar, and low-nutrient-content food out of convenience and simply not knowing any better, or just not taking into account the major drawbacks of poor snacking habits. The best solution to body-damaging snacking - in a nutshell – is to…

prepare ahead of time!

Follow these guidelines for energy boosting, body-building and mood enhancing snacks that will be a positive influence for you and everyone else in your life:

1. Only buy packaged snacks **after you have looked at the ingredient list** and determined that there are no added preservatives, sugar, artificial flavors or any long ingredient names that you can't pronounce or aren't familiar with. It a

general rule that anything with more than 5 ingredients is not likely to be a great choice either

2. **Eat raw and fresh produce whenever possible.** Consuming mostly organic is a good rule as well, but since price is certainly a factor for some, try to at least get the organic fruits and vegetables on the list below that are most effected by pesticides.

Avoid Chemical Laden Produce & Buy the Organic Option of:
Apples **Bell Peppers** **Blueberries** **Celery Cherries** **Imported grapes Kale** **Nectarines** **Peaches** **Potatoes Spinach** **Strawberries**

If you would like a handy chart for your fridge and wallet you can get this one-pager here:

http://www.prevention.com/pdf/DirtyDozen_ShoppingList.pdf

It provides you with the list of what to buy organic and what fruits and vegetables are safe to buy conventional.

3. **Get creative with your snacking.** Cook up some healthy recipes and separate into snack size servings so they are ready to munch on at a moment's notice or grab on the way out the door.

4. Are you a chip fanatic? **Resist the conventional potato chips that are high in salt and deep fried**. You'll be amazed at how tasty and crunchy your own homemade potato chips are! Thinly slice one simple potato (best done with a slicing blade in a hand slicer or food processor to make appropriately thin) and place a batch in between 2 pieces of parchment paper in the microwave. Season with a sprinkle of salt or other herbs and cook for 5-7 minutes, until they are lightly browned.

5. **Fancy up your fruits and vegetables with savory dips and tangy sauces.** This will provide lots of variety along with a treat for your sweet tooth. Make your own so you can control what's in them. Peanut butter (with just peanuts), slightly heated is tasty treat with various fruits and vegetables.

6. **Keep a supply of natural raw nuts around you all the time.** Don't worry about the fat content in nuts, it's the good fat your body soaks up and uses to your benefit. You can be more concerned about over consuming high-carb foods like

wheat products, potatoes and rice. Plus, nuts are packed with protein, antioxidants and the body friendly fat: omega-3 fatty acids!

7. **Dedicate your snacking to fruits and vegetables**. Many people find it difficult to consume the required amount of fruits and vegetables the body craves to function at its peak performance. Make one of your goals to only snack on fruit and vegetable based snacks.

The Healthy Art of Juicing

Another snacking wonder is extracting the juice from those so important fruits and vegetables. Juicing is an optimum way to be sure to get a healthy dose of your recommended daily intake. Although juicing doesn't provide the fiber that eating the whole food would do, you are getting a concentrated form of the vitamins, minerals and phytonutrients that are better absorbed directly into your system. *Don't cut out eating whole produce altogether*, but use juicing as a power packed snack that ups your intake of the right foods and allows you to have a nutrient filled drink in an efficient manner.

A common reason that juicing is so popular is the ability to consume vegetables and fruits that aren't quite so enjoyable eating otherwise. Mix those undesirable with some of the more appealing tastes and you'll hardly even notice the spinach and kale sliding down with the apples and carrots.

Raw is always best.

Although, you can still feel good about adding some cooked vegetables with your meal, a cooked vegetable will always have a lower amount of those vital and sensitive micronutrients when the food is heated. With the simple process of juicing you get high-nutrient drink custom made to your liking.

A note of caution about juicing fruits: Along with the high quality nutrients comes a high sugar content, so limit fruit in your juice mixes so you're not spiking your insulin levels.

Keeping yourself informed of the good, the bad, and the ugly of food and drink will keep you one step ahead of any diet blunders. You will save yourself from additional risk of developing a wide range of diseases and disorders by gathering lots of information about the specific foods that will provide the optimum fuel for you to get your body operating at peak performance. The more you know the better life will go, and your body will be an excellent example of your knowledge in action.

BUILDING FITNESS

Exercising doesn't have to be a high-cardio session or a sweat-filled weight lifting experience. Approaching your health from a fitness point of view just has to include activity, and the more variety you have, the more likely it is that you'll actually look forward to physical activity. So to first lay the foundation for an active life let's go over the benefits of exercise and how it can improve several areas of your life.

- Getting the most obvious benefit out of the way, **being active is a surefire way to reduce weight or maintain a healthy weight**. Moving burns calories, even the most casual type of movement burns calories so you're sure to get that benefit no matter what your mobility or physical condition.

- Regular physical activity will help you **mange or greatly reduce the risk of contracting various health conditions and diseases**. A few examples of these disorders and diseases are: type 2 diabetes, depression, heart disease, certain types of cancer, osteoporosis, stroke and arthritis.

- As mentioned in the above point, exercising is a form of treatment for depression, it also helps to get you feeling happier and more relaxed. Various brain chemicals are released by exercise that lifts your spirit and gives you a more positive outlook.

- Once you get over the fact that you don't always feel like you have the energy to be active, you can embrace the reality that after exercising (especially when providing your body with the appropriate fuel) **you will feel more energetic**. As well, you'll have a long-term flow of energy when you are increasing your heart rate on a daily basis.

- Have trouble sleeping? Exercise to the rescue! **Getting active regularly promotes a quicker and deeper sleep** when completed at least 4-5 hours before bedtime.

- Here's the relationship booster: **regular physical activity promotes a happier sex life**. Various aspects come into play for this benefit. The energy boost will get you feeling in the mood and all those feel good hormones released during exercise (endorphins, dopamine, adrenaline, and serotonin) work synergistically to make you feel happy and confident which relates to an increased libido.

- Of course there's the buff, toned body and greater range ofmotion that you'll enjoy all throughout the day.

Physical Activity That Fits You

Outside of the going-to-the-gym-routine and joining in guided fitness classes there are several ways to get more exercise in your day.

Incorporating just a couple of these exercising examples will not only help you reap the benefits of exercise, but also create a lifestyle full of fun, new experiences and a deeper inner awareness.

Getting your exercise in the great outdoors has the added benefit of soaking in the natural surroundings. There are several easy ways to incorporate cardiovascular activities that you can do with little or no equipment and spontaneously start right away.

> *Running or walking* – a brisk walk can be just as beneficial as running so don't go for the high-impact option thinking it's the healthier way. Apart from maybe needing some shoes with good support, especially for running, these two activities are possible for anyone, at any time, without any extra equipment. Also try to create a longer walk for yourself by parking far away from your intended destination or go for a quick walk as you're going about your day – just for the health of it!

> *Biking* – most people already have a bike, but if not, it's a great investment and you don't need to go top-quality. Any bike that you can ride will do. Making the choice to ride your bike instead of taking your vehicle out is a popular way to get some exercise while going about your daily activities. Great for the environment too!

> *Skiing/snowshoeing* – for those that get to experience snowy climates, taking up some type of activity that is dependent on the snow is not only good for your health

but also helps you to not dread the winter's negative side effects so much.

➢ *Stair climbing* – If you have a set of stairs in your home, you can use these for exercising purposes, but the concept can also be used to just naturally add some extra physical activity to your day by choosing to take a flight of stairs instead of an elevator or taking advantage of a quick exercise by traveling an outdoor set of stairs.

➢ *Jumping on a trampoline* – an exercise trampoline is a very small investment but provides an easy source of exercise. This is a simple way to add ten minutes here and ten minutes there of activity. You can run, jump with two feet or alternating feet, spin and jump, jump-kick and lot more fun high-cardio activity without the high-impact.

➢ *Skipping* – not just for children, skipping provides a low-cost easy way to get an excellent cardio workout that provides a number of benefits like high calorie burning, improved coordination, strengthening of core muscles and enhanced bone density.

Along with cardio activity, you will want to incorporate some flexibility and strength training exercise to get the full healthy effects of a well-cared for body.

> *Yoga/Pilates* – You can attend classes with a Yoga or Pilates instructor, which could be beneficial now and again, but these are compatible exercises to do in the comfort of your own home. Get a video that you can follow along with or do your own sequence of positions after you get familiar with some of the moves. Although there are some differences between Yoga and Pilates, they both focus on increasing flexibility and muscle tone and you can ease your way into more challenging moves.

> *Bodyweight Training* – this type of exercise uses the weight and movement of your own body to tone and build strong muscles. A couple of well-known examples would be push-ups, squats, crunches and lunges. There are many different exercises that are considered bodyweight training, which allows for variety and numerous options to choose exercises best for your goals and preferences.

➢ *Weight Lifting* – done with free weights, this is similar to bodyweight training with the addition of even more possibilities for exercises and a greater ability to build stronger muscles. Having just a couple of different sized weights allows you to experience a wide range of weight bearing exercises while not having to own a lot of equipment.

➢ *Flexibility Training* – also referred to as stretching, that basic natural bodily function that feels great after a sleep or sitting for long periods of time, is also a key fitness principal to a healthy body. By stretching your body, you are extending and lengthening your joints which increases flexibility and results in better control of all your movements throughout the day. Yoga and Pilates are considered a form of flexibility training but for a different approach and wider array of exercises you can perform a basic calf stretch, hamstring stretch, shoulder stretch, etc. The image below shows a stretching routine that is a great option to do *before* high intensity cardio exercises or *after* any type of physical activity when the muscles are warm and more easily lengthened.

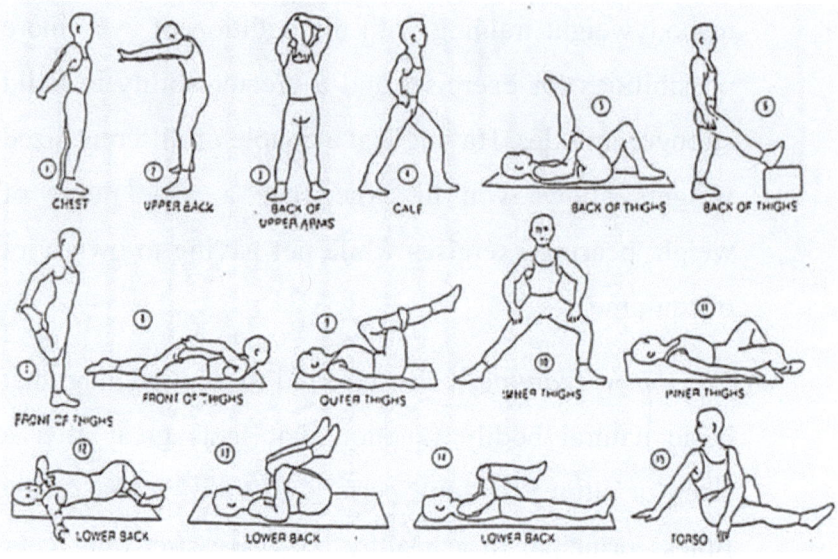

CHEST   UPPER BACK   BACK OF UPPER ARMS   CALF   BACK OF THIGHS   BACK OF THIGHS   FRONT OF THIGHS   FRONT OF THIGHS   OUTER THIGHS   INNER THIGHS   INNER THIGHS   LOWER BACK   LOWER BACK   LOWER BACK   TORSO

Ideally, your body would love it if you gave it at least 30 minutes of cardiovascular activity every day along with a 10-20 minute strength training session and a lengthening flexibility routine of another 10 minutes. If you commit to this you'll see and feel the great results of your commitment on the inside and out. However, this can also be a goal to achieve as you're making slow progress towards a health-focused lifestyle. To start off your gradual progress towards a physically active life, commit to 10 minutes of cardio exercise 4-5 times a week. Perhaps you'll have a few days where you'll gladly take that high energy walk for 30 minutes or have so much fun leaping, hopping and spinning on a trampoline that you didn't even notice 20 minutes go by. Those will be little bonuses and it'll feel great and give you a boost to see how easily you can get fit and feel great, but keep your 10 minute goal for a whole week and each week, or even every couple of weeks, increase your time until you reach the minimum 30 minutes

By all means do more if that's what feels right to you! Best not to get obsessed over exercise – there is more to life, after all – but experiment with different exercises and you'll be pleasantly surprised to find a few activities that you genuinely enjoy doing. Because you really should be doing what you enjoy in every area of your life. Sure, everyone has a few tasks they'd rather not do, but those tasks shouldn't take up much time and shouldn't relate to you achieving a holistic state of health.

GETTING THERE: TARGETS AND OBJECTIVES

You know that taking care of your health is important. Creating the right mindset is the initial step to embarking on a change for the better that will allow you to prepare for the emotional struggle that is often associated with a lifestyle adjustment. To complement all that mental preparation you will secure your success by setting milestones of achievement that will be a motivational tool to help you reach your ultimate goal of an active and healthy life.

As the old saying goes 'talk is cheap' and you can talk about what you *want to do* to 20 people and still turn up short on your objectives. It's not necessarily because you are not genuine in your conversations but merely because creating a plan on paper creates a visual aspect to your goals that your subconscious can internalize to a greater depth. That's what you want- depth and sincerity to your desires not just a verbal expression.

46

Create a plan, follow it through and gauge your progress along the way.

A very common system for setting goals uses the acronym SMART as outlined below:

Specific	Define your goal in a short direct statement
Measurable	Be sure your goal is something that you can determine when it's completed i.e. "I will lose 10 pounds…" as opposed to "I will lose weight"
Attainable	This is the warning against setting a goal that would be very difficult for you to achieve. The purpose of setting goals is to assist you in achieving a healthy life, so you want to achieve lots of morale-boosting smaller goals to work your way to the big one.
Rewarding	Make your goal an appealing reward that you can be excited about and not an obligatory response to a friend's suggestion.
Time-bound	Set a time for completion. Don't agonize over an unreached goal in the predicted time. It's not a matter of completing a goal in the length of time set or don't do it at all. If the time comes and you still haven't attained your goal then just set a new date and adjust other components of the goal if desired.

While looking at the general goal of improving your health, look at what little things you need to do to achieve that.

Are there some bad habits that you need to get rid of? Do you need to learn more about nutrition?

Are you aware of the exercises that are most effective for your body type?

These are just a few questions to get you thinking of the various small goals that you can set for yourself. Organize your goals in a way that allows you to complete the simplest tasks first and then move on to the more difficult achievements after you've built up some motivation from your past successfully attained goals. Look over the sample set of nutrition goals below to get in the mindset of self-analysis to best describe your personal goals.

GOAL #1	Read *The Juicing Book* by Stephen Blauer by May 25th
	Progress & Notes:
GOAL #2	Prepare raw vegetables on Sundays and Wednesdays to use for juicing and snacking
	Progress & Notes: *progress most important for this type of goal. Record every time you do this on a Sunday and Wednesday until you have at least 3 consecutive weeks of completing the specifics of this type of goal*
GOAL #3	Buy only natural (unprocessed) meats by June 2nd
	Progress & Notes:

Group your goals into different areas of health so that you have nutrition goals, fitness goals, and emotional health goals (focused on relaxation, personal time and mental stability). Use the first few pages, or the last few pages of your health journal to record all your goals and also include a section for long-term goals that you would like to achieve in 1-3 years.

An excellent online resource to plan and track your goals is at http://trello.com. This site is designed as a project planner or task organizer, and is very effective to plan and track goals. There are several ways you can organize on this platform, so play around with it to work out the most effective process for you. This is very useful for your personal goal setting and implementation, but the other awesome feature of Trello is the option to share certain boards or organizations with other Trello members. With this feature you can add your accountability partner to your health goals board or organization and they can check in on your progress and comment. Hopefully you are able to connect with someone who is working towards some healthier living as well and you can share your planning and progress with each other.

Personal goal setting helps you to choose where you want to go in your life. Along with creating your health goals you can use this same process of setting and implementing goals in any area of your life. Thinking about your ideal future and planning out the steps to get there is a powerful method that provides a great deal of personal satisfaction and fulfillment and helps you realize more about yourself to make the most of your life.

The first page of *Fat to Firm at Any Age*, a Prevention Health Book, lists 'The 10 Commandments' of their Fat-to-Firm Program that lays out some basic concepts of healthy living and is a good indicator of what kind of goals you can be creating (or not creating) for yourself.

1. Thou shalt never diet again.
2. Thou shalt tally pleasure, not calories.
3. Thou shalt eat early and often.
4. Thou shalt escape personal fat traps.
5. Thou shalt exercise smarter, not harder.
6. Thou shalt work with your body type, not against it.
7. Thou shalt nourish your body *and* soul.
8. Thou shalt do what works for you.
9. Thou shalt forgive thyself for "mistakes."
10. Thou shalt celebrate small successes.

SETTING A HEALTHY EXAMPLE

When you've taken all the right steps to intentionally change your body for the better you'll be able to deal with the hurdles and set-backs with a much calmer mind. Target your expectations with a thorough plan and well organized agenda to put your best foot forward and enjoy the process along the way. All your effort and enthusiasm will pay off in your own life as well as affecting everyone you come in contact with. Loved ones, acquaintances, and casual contacts will be influenced by your dedication and genuine interest in taking care of yourself.

With a renewed perspective on health and an obvious growth of knowledge you will be someone that can offer guidance and compassion to others from your own experience. Being a good role model for those special people in your life can be motivation enough to stick with the battle of change. While you'll start out with many questions, possible frustrations and an air of uncertainty, you can feel confident that will soon pass and you can be one of the leaders of healthy living.

Spread the Happiness of Healthy Living

"Never underestimate the power of a small group of committed people to change the world. In fact, it is the only thing that ever has."
Margaret Mead

Through your individual choice to be healthier, whatever your underlying reasons are, you could be quite a committed example to many people around you. Hopefully your positive example will rub off and start a chain reaction – a paradigm shift - to a better food supply and smarter generations that can alter the common thought that food is less important than it really is.

At one time in our human history people could only source the 'natural' foods as they're classified as today. The hunter-gatherer diet of the past was completely plant-based with the addition of a meat product now and again. The body functions best when it's not overwhelmed with foreign substances that it's forced to process – not for any use by the body, but just as a waste product. The state of the filtering system of the human body is overused in the majority of cases. This constant strain from the numerous toxins entering the body through food, drink and our environment takes its toll in various ways through disease, discomfort, mental instability and other physical impairments.

Be the change that many people want to see in the world. Change can be hard, but change for the better is so rewarding and self-gratifying that one can hardly help inspiring others to feel better, treat the environment better and experience the paradigm shift that is slowly catching throughout the world.

At this point it's mainly just about you feeling good and getting your body in better shape. Your internal drive, planning and learning about a natural way to live will keep you on track and then, when you achieve some of your goals, you're going to subconsciously be impressing your new-found perspective on others.

Be prepared to be admired.

Be prepared to be a mentor and be asked for your input. You may be a humble soul and reading this with a bit of uncertainty, assuming that your desire to be a better person isn't that big of a deal for other people, but it really is. You can probably figure that your immediate family will be affected, if only because they will be undoubtedly privy to your efforts.

Perhaps you were inspired by someone you knew that was taking control of their lives and creating a healthier and happier lifestyle? You can surely imagine that you will be a positive role model for any number of people in your circle of friends and family. It's a given and hopefully it's a thought that you can use as motivation to never give up on the health-focused life. It's no secret that the masses tend to favor unhealthy choices otherwise we would see a number of corporations no longer operating. We are creatures of habit though and we tend to take on the ideals and perspective of those that surround us, whether it's from the media or individuals.

The world simply needs better role models and lots more of them to spread the perspective of a more enjoyable life.

Hey, if you're not quite up to the task of encouraging a healthy life for others at the beginning of your path to health, that's OK. I guarantee that you'll feel up to it after you experience a better way to be and you're well established in new healthy life!

"The world is a dangerous place to live; not because of the people who are evil, but because of the people who don't do anything about it."

Albert Einstein

CONCLUSION

Are you up to the task?

It's one of the most important decisions you'll make for yourself. Taking on more healthier habits will effectively allow you to live to your true potential and not be held back by poor health and all the negative side-effects that come with it. As you probably know, you don't have to be diagnosed with a debilitating disease to have poor health affect you. You can be effected by difficult to control emotions, lack of energy, disinterest in being active (which is contrary to the natural human condition to be striving, achieving and creating), and a myriad of other symptoms that just make life difficult.

Some profound words from Isaac Asimov (1920-1992 American author and professor of biochemistry):

"It has been my philosophy of life that difficulties vanish when faced boldly."

Boldly face the difficult task of striving for better health. Life can be a struggle but as many have said, 'at least I've got my health'. It just seems to make life so much more difficult when you have to face challenges involving your health. If you already have health issues then you know best that making healthier choices is so important right now. Don't ever doubt that you are able to effectively manage any health issues by treating yourself with the basic medicine of proper nutrition, exercise and spiritual nourishment.

In the words of Hippocrates...

"Let food be thy medicine and medicine be thy food."

Words from long ago still speak true today. Eating the right foods and avoiding harmful foods will allow your body to heal itself. Although this is not a statement to discredit the treatment of your doctor, this is a statement to empower you to take an active role in your health, whether you are dealing with disease or disorders or deeply desire to avoid them.

Now equipped with knowledge and advice to take you through this process of change with a focus on health, you may soon find that there are other areas of your life that you want to see some change in.

Becoming the Person You Really Want To Be

It's simple to say you want to change, but it takes persistence and motivation to make that change happen. You are a product of your upbringing and it's not always good stuff that surrounded you. In fact, there will often be something that has been an influence from others that may have worked for them but it's not working for you. The influence of others isn't just from childhood when we are all highly impressionable, it also comes from fellow adults that you value and unconsciously adopt their perspective.

Decide what other things aren't working for you in your life and focus more on how you want to be instead of trying to figure out how you're going to stop being a certain way. A few simple questions will help you define what is important for you and what to strengthen in your life:

> ➢ What are your priorities concerning career, family, social activities and personal growth?

➢ What character traits do you admire in others that you would like to have yourself?

➢ What people make you feel good when you're around them and add value to your life?

Write down your priorities, the character traits you want to develop, and the people that you should surround yourself with. With these answers you can start to determine what other things you need to work on to make progress on your path to complete personal growth.

To make those changes and be that better and wiser person, daily attention is needed. Spend some time each day thinking about what you'd do, what you'd say and how you would react in various situations being the person you'd really like to be.

Envision your life the way you want it.

This doesn't have to be one 10-20 minute stretch, but if you find that days are going by and you are forgetting this important activity, then make an appointment with yourself each day to do this. A less regimented attempt would be to have these thoughts several times in a day when you have the opportunity to let your mind wander. This is a casual way to 'trick' yourself into change. Jot thoughts down in your health journal, share them with your accountability partner and bring them up in conversation with anyone in your life. Personal growth in every area of your life is a lifelong endeavour that is never truly over. Our childhood is full new experiences that shape and form our personalities – some good, some not so good.

Once we become adults and accountable for our actions, it can become apparent that there are a few things that we grew up with that doesn't work. Part of maturing is realizing what we need to change and taking on the arduous task of making that change happen. You never have to accept anything about yourself that you are not happy with and you have the power to make that change happen – even if it's something that's been engrained in you for years.

Make a plan, break free and take action!

You're making a decision to be free.

To be free of unhealthy information

To be free of constricting thoughts

To be free of limited nutrition

To be free of inactivity

To be free of purposeless days

To be free of an uninspiring life

To be free of ignorance when it comes to your health

Printed by Libri Plureos GmbH in Hamburg,
Germany